5-INGRED
RENAL DIET

Low Sodium and Low Potassium Recipes to Control Your Kidney Disease

Lara Benson

work can be in any fashion deemed liable for any hardship or damages that may befall them after undertaking information described herein.

Additionally, the information in the following pages is intended only for informational purposes and should thus be thought of as universal. As befitting its nature, it is presented without assurance regarding its prolonged validity or interim quality. Trademarks that are mentioned are done without written consent and can in no way be considered an endorsement from the trademark holder.

TABLE OF CONTENTS

Introduction

The Renal Diet focuses primarily on supporting kidney health because in doing so, you'll improve many other aspects of your health, as well. It can also be customized to fit all levels of kidney disease, from early stages and minor infections to more significant renal impairment and dialysis. Preventing the later stages is the primary goal, though reaching this stage can still be treated with careful consideration of your dietary choices. In addition to medical treatment, the diet provides a way for you to gain control over your health and progression.

Benefits of Renal Diet

The role of any diet for kidney disease, therefore, is very important as eating certain foods with varying levels of these minerals can either improve or worsen renal function. Specifically, the renal diet includes the following benefits:

Decreased fluid buildup in kidneys and other organs Mineral balance

Regulated blood pressure

All these three major benefits will help ease many symptoms of the disease and even limit dependency on certain drugs, e.g., diuretics, which may often lead to side effects when abused.

Diabetes and heart disease patients who also suffer from some type of kidney failure may also benefit from the renal diet as these problems are interconnected, and factors that influence one disorder, e.g., diet, will influence the other and vice versa. Therefore, if you are diagnosed with decreased kidney function, a renal diet will help you keep your kidney activity levels stable and help you avoid dialysis—which is the final and most difficult stage of renal failure and may put your health at serious risk.

A proper renal diet plan that is low in phosphorus, potassium, and sodium can slow down the progression of the renal disease and control the accompanying symptoms that often come with it, such as elevated blood pressure and mineral imbalance.

Foods to Eat

Cauliflower: It is enriched with anti-inflammatory compounds like insoles and is an excellent source of fiber

Blueberries: These sweet berries contain antioxidants called anthocyanin, which help protect against heart disease, certain cancers, cognitive decline, and diabetes...

Red grapes: are delicious as well as deliver plenty of nutrition in a small package. They were rich in vitamin C; contain antioxidants called flavonoids, which show characteristics of reducing inflammation...

Egg whites: egg yolks are very nutritious, containing high amounts of phosphorus, therefore, diverting attention to egg whites, and being a better choice for people following a renal diet. People who are experiencing dialysis treatment have higher protein needs but need to limit phosphorus...

Buckwheat: is an exception with high nutrition concentration, providing B vitamins, magnesium, iron, and fiber.

Garlic: It is a source of manganese, vitamin C, and vitamin B6, which also contains sulfur compounds having anti-inflammatory properties.

Olive oil: is a phosphorus-free option for people suffering from kidney disease. A significant chunk of fat in olive oil is a monounsaturated fat called oleic acid, which has anti-inflammatory properties. Monounsaturated fats, being stable at high temperatures, make olive oil a fruitful choice for cooking.

Cabbage: it has vitamin K, vitamin C, and many B vitamins and **minerals. It is low in potassium, phosphorus, and sodium**

Onions are a sodium-free flavor to renal-diet dishes. Onions, being applauded with vitamin C, manganese, and B complex, and prebiotic fibers help keep your digestive system safe and sound by feeding beneficial gut bacteria.

Foods to Avoid

1. **Canned Foods:** including soups, vegetables, and beans, are low in cost but contain high amounts of sodium due to salt's addition to increasing its life. One more way is to drain or rinse canned foods, such as canned beans and tuna.

2. **Brown Rice:** is a higher concentration of potassium and phosphorus than its white rice counterpart. One cup of already cooked brown rice possesses about 150 mg of phosphorus and 154 mg of potassium,

3. **Bananas:** are high potassium content, low in sodium, and provide 422 mg of potassium per banana. It might disturb your daily balanced potassium intake to 2,000 mg

4. **Pineapples:** contain less potassium than other tropical fruits and can be a more suitable alternative.

5. **Whole-Wheat Bread:** White bread is recommended instead of whole-wheat varieties for individuals with kidney disease because it has phosphorus and potassium.

6. **Oranges and Orange Juice:** are enriched with vitamin C content and potassium. An orange of 184 g. provides 333 mg. of potassium, and one orange juice cup provides 473 mg. of potassium.

7. **Processed Meats:** are the cause of chronic diseases and are unhealthy due to the content of preservatives. Processed

meats are those which might be salted, or dried, or packaged in cans

8. **Potatoes and sweet potatoes:** like potatoes and sweet potatoes, some of the high-potassium foods could also be soaked or leached to lessen the concentration of potassium contents.

9. **Packaged, Instant, and Processed foods, instant, and pre-made meals:** are the most heavily processed and contain a higher sodium concentration.

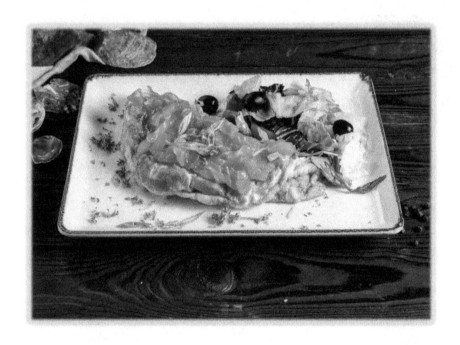

Renal Diet Recipes

Fried Eggs, Bacon & Asparagus

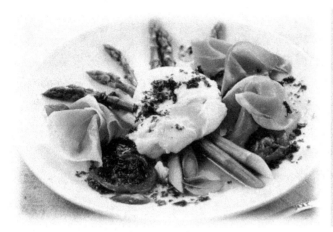

Time required:
12 minutes

_____

Servings: 02

INGREDIENTS	STEPS FOR COOKING

INGREDIENTS

2 medium eggs
4 asparagus springs, trimmed
2 slices of streaky bacon, cut into square bits
½ tbsp. Chives chopped
¼ tsp. Salt
⅛ tsp. ground pepper

STEPS FOR COOKING

1. Heat a skillet over medium heat and cook the bacon bits until nice and crispy (approx. 3 minutes). Leave their fat and take off the heat.

2. Add the asparagus spears and cover the pan. Let cook covered for 5 minutes or until slightly softened.

3. Add the eggs, cover, and cook for another couple of minutes or until the egg whites are set. Check if the yolk is done to your likeness.

4. Season with the chives, salt, and pepper, and serve.

Oatmeal & Berry Pancakes

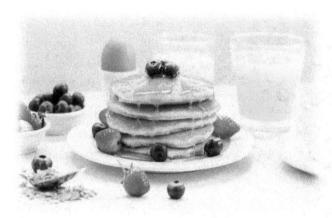

Time required:
8 minutes

Servings: 04

INGREDIENTS	STEPS FOR COOKING

INGREDIENTS

½ cup (40g) of rolled oats
⅓ cup (80ml) rice milk 1 tbsp. Of honey
¼ cup (25g) blueberries Cooking spray

STEPS FOR COOKING

1. Blend all the ingredients in a food processor until you end up with a creamy paste.

2. Spray a small skillet with cooking spray and spoon off the mixture in small circle parts. Use the spoon to disperse the mixture in the pan's center, making small round pancakes (around 3-4 inches in diameter). Cook for 1 minute on one side and then flip with a spatula.

3. Repeat all the above steps to finish the mixture.

Mexican Style Burritos

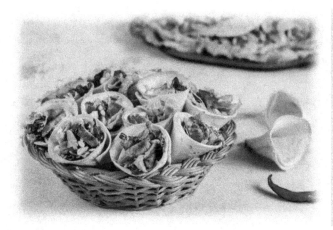

Time required:
25 minutes

Servings: 02

INGREDIENTS

2 corn tortillas

¼ cup red onion, chopped

½ red chili, deseeded and chopped

2 eggs

1 lime, juiced

1 tbsp. cilantro, chopped

¼ cup red bell peppers, chopped

1 tbsp. olive oil

STEPS FOR COOKING

1. Place the tortillas in a broiler on medium heat for 1–2 minutes on each side or until lightly toasted.

2. Remove and keep the broiler on.

3. Heat the oil in a skillet and sauté the onion, chili, and bell peppers for 5–6 minutes, or until soft.

4. Crack the eggs over the top of the onions and peppers.

5. Place the skillet under the broiler for 5–6 minutes or until the eggs are cooked.

6. Serve half the eggs and vegetables on top of each tortilla and sprinkle with the cilantro and lime juice to serve.

Arugula Eggs with Chili Peppers

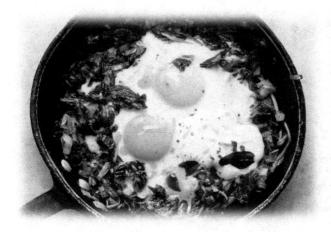

Time required:
15 minutes

Servings: 04

INGREDIENTS	STEPS FOR COOKING
2 cups arugula, chopped 3 eggs, beaten ½ chili pepper, chopped 1 tbsp. butter 1 oz. Parmesan, grated	1. Toss the butter in the skillet and melt it. 2. Add the arugula and sauté it over medium heat for 5 minutes. Stir it from time to time. 3. Meanwhile, mix up the Parmesan, chili pepper, and eggs. 4. Pour the egg mixture over the arugula and scramble well. 5. Cook for 5 minutes more over medium heat.

French Toast with Applesauce

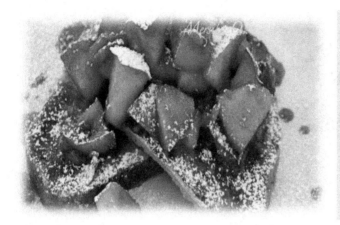

Time required:
25 minutes

_____

Servings: 06

INGREDIENTS

¼ cup unsweetened
applesauce
½ cup almond milk
1 teaspoon ground
cinnamon
2 eggs
2 tablespoon white
sugar

STEPS FOR COOKING

1. Mix well applesauce, sugar, cinnamon, almond milk and eggs in a mixing bowl.

2. Soak the bread, one by one into applesauce mixture until wet.

3. On medium fire, heat a nonstick skillet greased with cooking spray.

4. Add soaked bread one at a time and cook for 2-3 minutes per side or until lightly browned.

5. Serve and enjoy.

Bagels Made Healthy

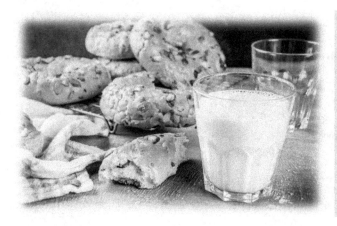

Time required:
35 minutes

Servings: 08

INGREDIENTS

2 teaspoon yeast
1 ¼ cups bread flour
2 cups whole wheat flour
2 tablespoons honey
1 ½ cups warm water
1 ½ tablespoon olive oil

STEPS FOR COOKING

1. In a bread machine, mix all ingredients, and then process on dough cycle.
2. Once done or end of cycle, create 8 pieces shaped like a flattened ball.
3. In the center of each ball, make a hole using your thumb then create a donut shape.
4. In a greased baking sheet, place donut-shaped dough then covers and let it rise about ½ hour.
5. Prepare about 2 inches of water to boil in a large pan.
6. In a boiling water, drop one at a time the bagels and boil for 1 minute, then turn them once.
7. Remove them and return them to baking sheet and bake at 350oF (175oC) for about 20 to 25 minutes until golden brown.

Grandma's Pancake Special

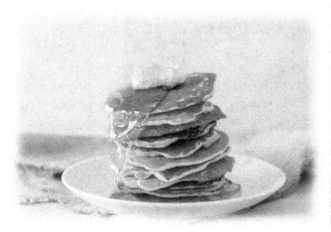

Time required:
20 minutes

Servings: 03

INGREDIENTS

1 cup almond milk
1 egg
2 teaspoons sodium free baking powder
2 tablespoons sugar
1 ¼ cups flour
1 tablespoon oil

STEPS FOR COOKING

1. Mix together all the dry ingredients such as the flour, sugar and baking powder.

2. Combine oil, almond milk and egg in another bowl. Once done, add them all to the flour mixture.

3. Make sure that as your stir the mixture, blend them together until slightly lumpy.

4. In a hot greased griddle, pour-in at least ¼ cup of the batter to make each pancake.

5. To cook, ensure that the bottom is a bit brown, then turn and cook the other side, as well.

Feta Mint Omelette

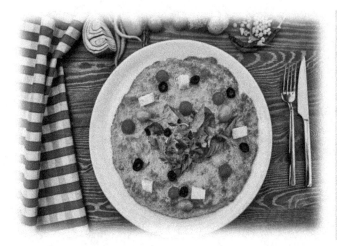

Time required:
15 minutes

Servings: 01

INGREDIENTS

3 eggs
1/4 cup fresh mint,
chopped
2 tbsp coconut milk
1/2 tsp olive oil
2 tbsp feta cheese,
crumbled
Pepper
Salt

STEPS FOR COOKING

1. In a bowl, whisk eggs with feta cheese, mint, milk, pepper, and salt.
2. Heat olive oil in a pan over low heat.
3. Pour egg mixture in the pan and cook until eggs are set.
4. Flip omelet and cook for 2 minutes more.
5. Serve and enjoy.

Breakfast Maple Sausage

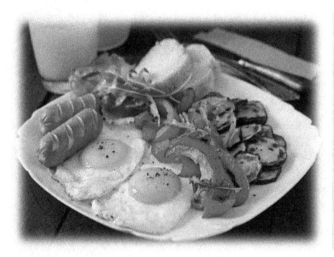

Time required:
15 minutes

Servings: 01

INGREDIENTS

3 eggs
1/4 cup fresh mint,
chopped
2 tbsp coconut milk
1/2 tsp olive oil
2 tbsp feta cheese,
crumbled
Pepper
Salt

STEPS FOR COOKING

1. In a bowl, whisk eggs with feta cheese, mint, milk, pepper, and salt.
2. Heat olive oil in a pan over low heat.
3. Pour egg mixture in the pan and cook until eggs are set.
4. Flip omelet and cook for 2 minutes more.
5. Serve and enjoy.

Chicken Egg Breakfast Muffins

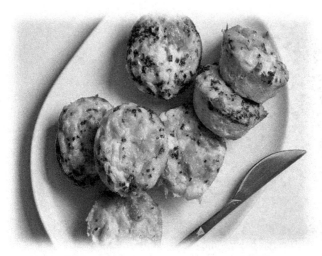

Time required:
25 minutes

Servings: 12

INGREDIENTS

10 eggs

1 cup cooked chicken, chopped

3 tbsp green onions, chopped

1/4 tsp garlic powder

Pepper Salt

STEPS FOR COOKING

1. Preheat the oven to 400 F.
2. Spray a muffin tray with cooking spray and set aside.
3. In a large bowl, whisk eggs with garlic powder, pepper, and salt.
4. Add remaining ingredients and stir well.
5. Pour egg mixture into the muffin tray and bake for 15 minutes.
6. Serve and enjoy.

Egg Drop Soup

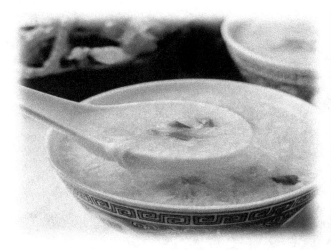

Time required:
15 minutes

Servings: 04

INGREDIENTS

¼ cup minced fresh chives

4 cups unsalted vegetable stock 4 whisked eggs

STEPS FOR COOKING

1. Pour unsalted vegetable stock into the oven set over high heat. Bring to a boil. Lower heat.

2. Pour in the eggs. Stir until ribbons form into the soup.

3. Turn off the heat immediately. The residual heat will cook eggs through.

4. Cool slightly before ladling the desired amount into individual bowls. Garnish with a pinch of parsley, if using.

5. Serve immediately.

Smoked Salmon and Poached Eggs on Toast

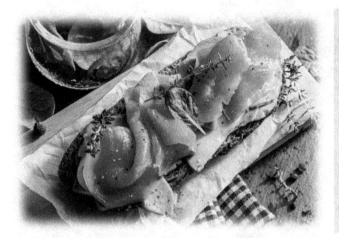

Time required:
25 minutes

Servings: 04

INGREDIENTS	STEPS FOR COOKING

INGREDIENTS

2 oz avocado smashed
2 slices of bread toasted
1/4 tsp freshly squeezed lemon juice
2 eggs
1 tbsp. Thinly sliced scallions
Pinch of kosher salt and cracked black pepper

STEPS FOR COOKING

1. Take a small bowl and then smash the avocado into it. Then, add the lemon juice and also a pinch of salt into the mixture. Then, mix it well and set aside.

2. After that, poach the eggs and toast the bread for some time. Once the bread is toasted, you will have to spread the avocado on both slices and after that, add the smoked salmon to each slice.

3. Thereafter, carefully transfer the poached eggs to the respective toasts. Add a splash of kikkoman soy sauce and some cracked pepper; then, just garnish with scallions and microgreens.

Warm Salmon

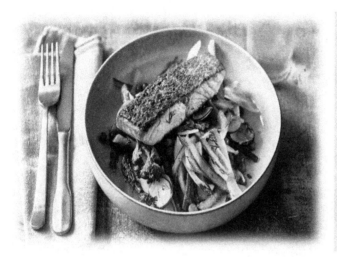

Time required:
35 minutes

Servings: 04

INGREDIENTS

400g baby new potato, halved
2 salmon fillets, skin on, (about 140g/5oz each)
small handful sundried tomato chopped
crushed juice 1/2 lemon
200g green beans
1 tbsp olive oil

STEPS FOR COOKING

1. Bring half of a large steamer to a boil, pour in the potatoes, then the salmon fillets, skin side down.

2. Cover and cook for 6-8 minutes until the salmon is cooked through, then set aside.

3. Cook the potatoes for another 5-8 minutes until tender, adding the beans for the last couple of minutes. Drain the vegetables, pour into a bowl. Also add the olives and tomatoes, flake the cooked salmon into pieces, discarding the skin.

4. Whisk the garlic, lemon and oil with some of the dressing, and dissolve with a few drops of water. Pour over the dressing, mix well and serve.

Berry Milk Smoothie

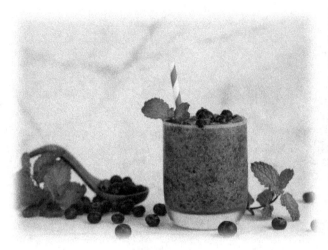

Time required:
5 minutes

Servings: 01

INGREDIENTS

½ cup fresh
blueberries
1 medium
cucumber, peeled
and sliced
½ cup fresh
strawberries
½ cup of almond
milk

STEPS FOR COOKING

1. First, begin by mixing all the ingredients into a blender jug.
2. Pulse it for 30 seconds until well blended.
3. Serve chilled.

Apple Cider

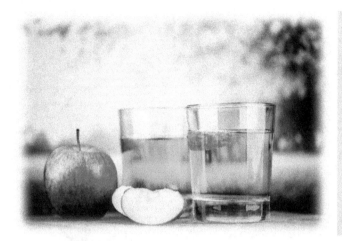

Time required:
15 minutes

Servings: 04

INGREDIENTS

4 cups apple cider
2 sticks cinnamon
3 cloves
5 allspice
2 cardamom pods,
crushed

STEPS FOR COOKING

1. Bring to a boil the cider into a pot.
2. Add the spices and softly cook for about 15 minutes.
3. Serve hot or cold and enjoy!

Cauliflower and Chive Soup

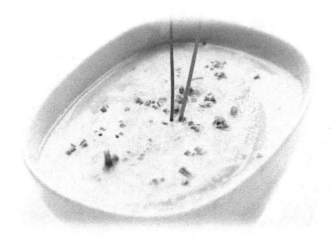

Time required:
35 minutes

Servings: 04

INGREDIENTS

2 tbsp extra-virgin olive oil –
½ sweet onion, chopped
2 garlic cloves, minced
2 cups Simple Chicken Broth
1 cauliflower head, broken into florets -
Freshly ground
4 tbsp (¼ cups) finely chopped chives

STEPS FOR COOKING

1. In a small stockpot over medium heat, heat the olive oil. Add the onion and cook, frequently stirring, for 3 - 5 minutes, until it begins to soften. Add the garlic and stir until fragrant.

2. Add the broth and cauliflower and bring to a boil. Reduce the heat and simmer until the cauliflower is tender about 15 minutes.

3. Transfer the soup in batches to a blender or food processor and purée until smooth or use an immersion blender. Return the soup to the pot, and season with pepper. Before serving, top each bowl with 1 tbsp of chives.

4. Cooking tip: If you're using a traditional blender, work in batches, and place a clean kitchen towel over the top of the lid as you blend to

INGREDIENTS	STEPS FOR COOKING
	prevent splashing hot soup. Fill the blender only to the safe-fill line, and be very cautious as you go, as hot liquids can be dangerous to work with.

Kidney-Friendly Chips

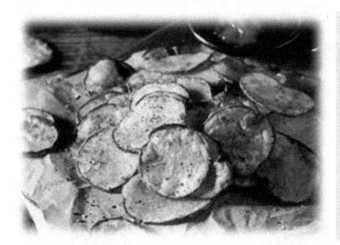

Time required:
60 minutes

Servings: 04

INGREDIENTS

*4 parsnips, peeled
and sliced*
*1 tbsp. extra virgin
olive oil*
1 tsp. black pepper
1 tsp. thyme
1 tsp. chili flakes

STEPS FOR COOKING

1. Heat oven to 375°f/190°c/gas mark 5.
2. Grease a baking tray with olive oil.
3. Add the parsnip slices in a thin layer.
4. Sprinkle over the thyme and chili slices and toss to coat.
5. Bake for 40-50 minutes (turning halfway through to ensure even crispiness!)

Spaghetti Squash Puree

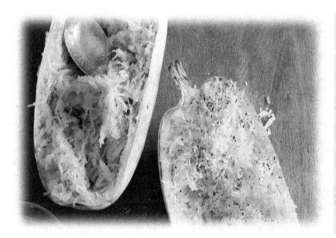

Time required:
25 minutes

—

Servings: 02

INGREDIENTS

1 spaghetti squash
(approx. 4 cups)
1 tsp. chili flakes
3 tbsp. parsley,
finely chopped
1 tbsp. extra virgin
olive oil

STEPS FOR COOKING

1. Pre-heat the oven to 375°f/190 °c/gas mark 5.
2. Cut squash in half lengthways.
3. Place each side into a large oven dish (skin up).
4. Pour half a cup of water into the dish.
5. Bake for 45 minutes or until tender.
6. Remove from the oven and allow cooling.
7. Flake with a fork to shred the flesh into a bowl.
8. Stir in the chili flakes, black pepper, parsley, and garlic cloves.
9. Blend in a food processor until smooth.
10. Serve on your favorite salad or with your favorite meat.

Cauliflower Cheese

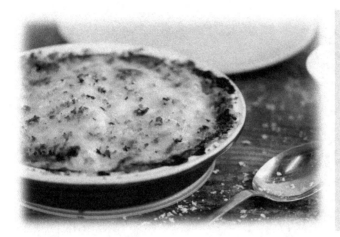

Time required:
45 minutes

Servings: 06

INGREDIENTS

1 large cauliflower (leaves cut off), broken into pieces
4 tbsp flour
500ml milk
100g (3½oz) strong cheddar, grated
3 tbsp breadcrumbs
50g (1¾oz) butter

STEPS FOR COOKING

1. Bring a big saucepan of water to the boil, add the cauliflower and cook for five minutes. Lift a slice to test, it should be cooked. Drain the cauliflower, then pour it into a dish that is ovenproof.

2. Heat the oven to 425 ° F / Gas 7 at 220 ° C (200 ° C fan).

3. Return the saucepan back to the heat and add the flour, butter, and milk. As the butter melts and the mixture comes to the boil, keep whisking quickly-the flour will vanish and the sauce will start thickening. Whisk for two minutes while the sauce bubbles and becomes smooth and thick. Turn the heat off, stir in much of the cheese and dump the cauliflower over it. Scatter over the remaining breadcrumbs and cheese.

INGREDIENTS	STEPS FOR COOKING
	4. In the oven, bake the cauliflower cheese for twenty minutes until it bubbles.
	5. Tip: Make enough for six servings, even if you need less as spare portions can be frozen before being baked.

Citrus Salad with Sour Cream

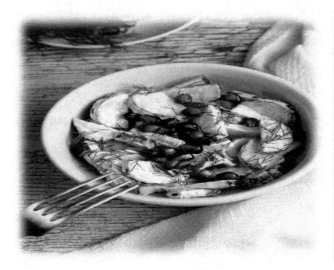

Time required:
15 minutes

Servings: 01

INGREDIENTS

50 ggrapefruit
50 g orange
25ml sour cream
lemon juice
salt

STEPS FOR COOKING

1. Peel the grapefruit and oranges and remove the inner hard skins or kernels from them.
2. Cut the fruit pulp into pieces, drizzle with lemon juice, lightly salt and pour over the cream.

Thai Cucumber Salad

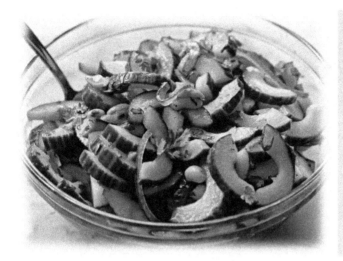

Time required:
15 minutes

Servings: 02

INGREDIENTS

¼ cup chopped
peanuts
¼ cup white sugar
¼ cup rice wine
vinegar
3 cucumbers
2 jalapeno peppers

STEPS FOR COOKING

1. Add all ingredients in a small basin
   and combine well.
2. Serve with dressing

Green Bean and Potato Salad

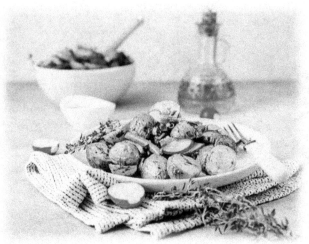

Time required:
10 minutes

Servings: 04

INGREDIENTS

½ cup basil
¾ lb. green beans
½ cup balsamic
vinegar
1 red onion
1 lb. red potatoes
¼ cup olive oil
1 tablespoon
mustard

STEPS FOR COOKING

1. Place potatoes in a pot with water and bring to a boil for 15-18 minutes or until tender
2. Thrown in green beans after 5-6 minutes
3. Drain and cut into cubes
4. In a bowl add all ingredients and mix well
5. Serve with dressing.

Grapes Jicama Salad

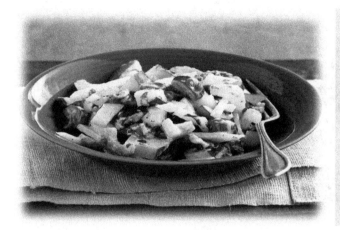

Time required:
5 minutes

Servings: 02

INGREDIENTS	STEPS FOR COOKING

1 jicama, peeled and sliced

1 carrot, sliced

½ medium red onion, sliced

1 ¼ cup seedless grapes

1/3 cup fresh basil leaves

1 tablespoon apple cider vinegar

½ tablespoon lime juice

1. Put all the salad ingredients into a suitable salad bowl.
2. Toss them well and refrigerate for 1 hour.
3. Serve.

Rutabaga Latkes

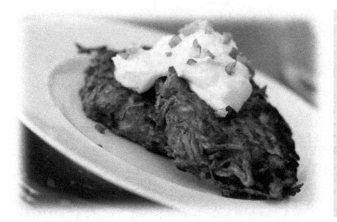

Time required:
25 minutes

Servings: 04

INGREDIENTS

1 teaspoon hemp
seeds
1 egg, beaten
7 oz rutabaga,
grated
½ teaspoon ground
paprika
2 tablespoons
coconut flour
1 teaspoon olive oil

STEPS FOR COOKING

1. Mix up together hemp seeds, ground black pepper, ground paprika, and coconut flour.

2. Then add grated rutabaga and beaten egg.

3. With the help of the fork combine together all the ingredients into the smooth mixture.

4. Preheat the skillet for 2-3 minutes over the high heat. Then reduce the heat till medium and add olive oil.

5. With the help of the fork, place the small amount of rutabaga mixture in the skillet. Flatten it gently in the shape of latkes.

6. Cook the latkes for 3 minutes from each side.

7. After this, transfer them in the plate and repeat the same steps with remaining rutabaga mixture.

Glazed Snap Peas

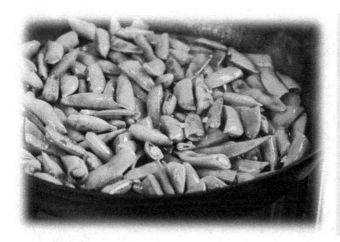

Time required:
5 minutes

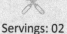

Servings: 02

INGREDIENTS	STEPS FOR COOKING
1 cup snap peas 2 teaspoon Erythritol 1 teaspoon butter, melted ¾ teaspoon ground nutmeg ¼ teaspoon salt 1 cup water, for cooking	1. Pour water in the pan. Add snap peas and bring them to boil. Boil the snap peas for 5 minutes over the medium heat. 2. Then drain water and chill the snap peas. 3. Meanwhile, whisk together ground nutmeg, melted butter, salt, and Erythritol. 4. Preheat the mixture in the microwave oven for 5 seconds. 5. Pour the sweet butter liquid over the snap peas and shake them well. The side dish should be served only warm.

Vegetable Masala

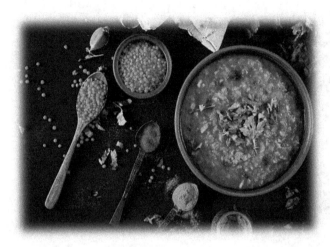

Time required:
35 minutes

Servings: 04

INGREDIENTS

2 cups green beans, chopped
1 cup white mushroom, chopped
¾ cup tomatoes, crushed
1 teaspoon minced garlic
1 teaspoon minced ginger
1 tablespoon garam masala
1 tablespoon olive oil
1 teaspoon salt

STEPS FOR COOKING

1. Line the tray with parchment and preheat the oven to 360F. Place the green beans and mushrooms in the tray.

2. Sprinkle the vegetables with crushed tomatoes, minced garlic and ginger, garam masala, olive oil, and salt.

3. Mix up well and transfer in the oven. Cook vegetable masala for 18 minutes.

Glazed Salmon

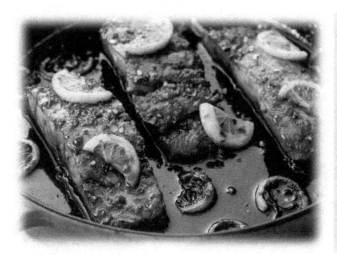

Time required:
20 minutes

Servings: 04

INGREDIENTS

4 (3-ounce) salmon
fillets

1 tablespoon of olive
oil

2 tablespoons of
honey

1 teaspoon of lemon
zest

½ teaspoon of black
pepper (ground), to
taste

½ scallion, chopped

STEPS FOR COOKING

1. Pat dry salmon with paper towels.
2. In a mixing bowl, add honey, lemon zest, and pepper.
3. Combine to mix well with each other.
4. Add salmon and coat evenly.
5. Take a medium saucepan or skillet, add oil. Heat over medium heat.
6. Add salmon and stir-cook until light brown and cooked well, about 8– 10 minutes.
7. Flip in between.
8. Serve warm with scallions on top.

Oregano Salmon with Crunchy Crust

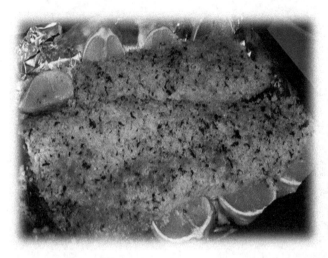

Time required:
2 hours

_____

Servings: 02

INGREDIENTS	STEPS FOR COOKING
8 oz of salmon fillet 2 tablespoons of panko bread crumbs 1 oz of Parmesan, grated 1 teaspoon of dried oregano 1 teaspoon of sunflower oil	1. In the mixing bowl combine together panko bread crumbs, Parmesan, and dried oregano. 2. Sprinkle the salmon with olive oil and coat in the breadcrumb's mixture. 3. After this, line the baking tray with baking paper. 4. Place the salmon in the tray and transfer in the preheated oven to 385o F. 5. Bake the salmon for 25 minutes.

Cajun Catfish

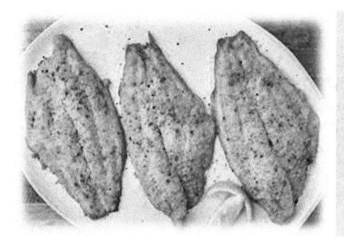

Time required:
20 minutes

Servings: 04

INGREDIENTS

*16 oz of catfish
steaks (4 oz each
fish steak)
1 tablespoon of
cajun spices
1 egg, beaten
1 tablespoon of
sunflower oil*

STEPS FOR COOKING

1. Pour sunflower oil in the skillet and preheat it until shimmering.
2. Meanwhile, dip every catfish steak in the beaten egg and coat in Cajun spices.
3. Place the fish steaks in the hot oil and roast them for 4 minutes from each side.
4. The cooked catfish steaks should have a light brown crust.

Poached Halibut in Orange Sauce

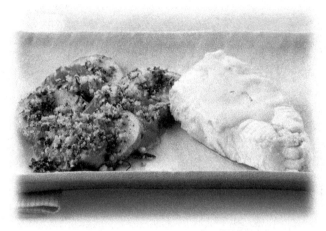

Time required:
25 minutes

Servings: 04

INGREDIENTS

1-pound halibut

1/3 cup butter

1 rosemary sprig

1 teaspoon honey

¼ cup of orange juice

1 teaspoon cornstarch

1 teaspoon salt

STEPS FOR COOKING

1. Put butter in the saucepan and melt it.
2. Add rosemary sprig.
3. Sprinkle the halibut with salt and ground black pepper.
4. Put the fish in the boiling butter and poach it for 4 minutes.
5. Meanwhile, pour orange juice in the skillet. Add honey and bring the liquid to boil.
6. Add cornstarch and whisk until the liquid will start to be thick.
7. Then remove it from the heat.
8. Transfer the poached halibut in the plate and cut it on 4.
9. Place every fish serving in the serving plate and top with orange sauce.

Poached Gennaro/Seabass with Red Peppers

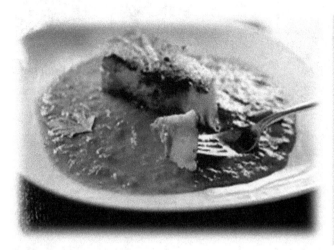

Time required:
55 minutes

Servings: 04

INGREDIENTS

2 red peppers, trimmed

11 oz Gennaro/seabass, trimmed

1 teaspoon salt

½ teaspoon ground black pepper

2 tablespoons butter

1 lemon

STEPS FOR COOKING

1. Remove the seeds from red peppers and cut them on the wedges.
2. Then line the baking tray with parchment and arrange red peppers in a layer.
3. Rub Gennaro/seabass with ground black pepper and salt and place it on the peppers.
4. Then add butter.
5. Cut the lemon on the halves and squeeze the juice over the fish.
6. Bake the fish for 40 minutes at 350F.

Salmon Balls with Cream Cheese

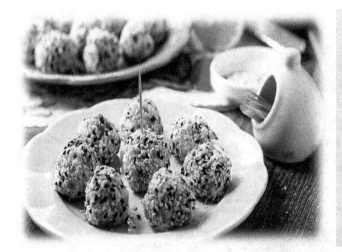

Time required:
35 minutes

Servings: 05

INGREDIENTS	STEPS FOR COOKING

INGREDIENTS

1-pound salmon fillet
2 teaspoons cream cheese
3 tablespoons panko breadcrumbs
½ teaspoon salt
1 oz Parmesan, grated
1 teaspoon dried oregano
1 tablespoon sunflower oil

STEPS FOR COOKING

1. Grind the salmon fillet and combine it together with cream cheese, panko breadcrumbs, salt, Parmesan, ground black pepper, and dried oregano.

2. Then make the small balls from the mixture and place them in the non-sticky tray.

3. Sprinkle the balls with sunflower oil and bake in the preheated to the 365F oven for 15 minutes. Flip the balls on another side after 10 minutes of cooking.

Lemon Broccoli

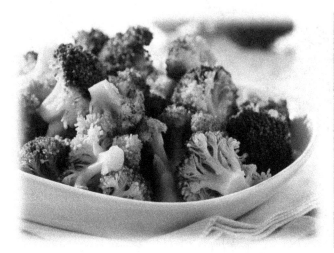

Time required:
35 minutes

Servings: 04

INGREDIENTS

2 heads broccoli, separated into florets

2 teaspoons extra virgin olive oil

1 teaspoon salt

½ teaspoon pepper

1 garlic clove, minced

½ teaspoon lemon juice

STEPS FOR COOKING

1. Pre-heat your oven to a temperature of 400 °F

2. Take a large-sized bowl and add broccoli florets with some extra virgin olive oil, pepper, sea salt and garlic

3. Spread the broccoli out in a single even layer on a fine baking sheet

4. Bake in your pre-heated oven for about 15-20 minutes until the florets are soft enough so that they can be pierced with a fork

5. Squeeze lemon juice over them generously before serving

6. Enjoy!

Eggplant Fries

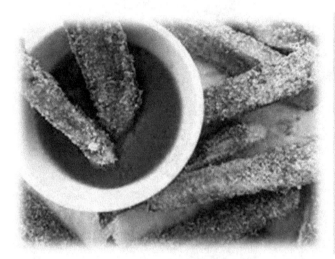

Time required:
25 minutes

Servings: 08

INGREDIENTS

2 eggs
2 cups almond flour
2 tablespoons
coconut oil, spray
2 eggplants, peeled
and cut thinly
Salt and pepper

STEPS FOR COOKING

1. Preheat your oven to 400 °F
2. Take a bowl and mix with salt and black pepper in it
3. Take another bowl and beat eggs until frothy
4. Dip the eggplant pieces into the eggs
5. Then coat them with the flour mixture
6. Add another layer of flour and egg
7. Then, take a baking sheet and grease with coconut oil on top
8. Bake for about 15 minutes.

Cauliflower Rice and Coconut

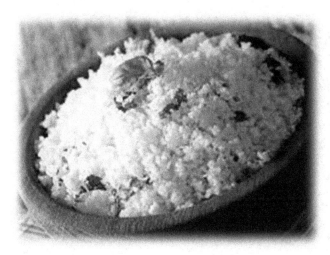

Time required:
45 minutes

Servings: 04

INGREDIENTS

3 cups cauliflower, riced

2/3 cups full-fat coconut almond milk

1-2 teaspoons sriracha paste

¼- ½ teaspoon onion powder

Salt as needed

Fresh basil for garnish

STEPS FOR COOKING

1. Take a pan and place it over medium-low heat

2. Add all of the ingredients and stir them until fully combined

3. Cook for about 5-10 minutes, making sure that the lid is on

4. Remove the lid and keep cooking until there's no excess liquid

5. Once the rice is soft and creamy, enjoy it!

Blistered Beans and Almond

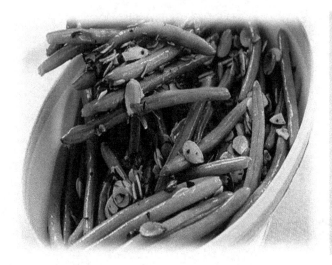

Time required:
35 minutes

Servings: 04

INGREDIENTS

1-pound fresh green beans, ends trimmed 1 ½ tablespoon olive oil
¼ teaspoon salt
1 ½ tablespoons fresh dill, minced
Juice of 1 lemon
¼ cup crushed almonds
Salt as needed

STEPS FOR COOKING

1. Preheat your oven to 400 °F
2. Add in the green beans with your olive oil and also the salt
3. Then spread them in one single layer on a large-sized sheet pan
4. Roast for 10 minutes and stir nicely, then roast for another 8-10 minutes
5. Remove it from the oven and keep stirring in the lemon juice alongside the dill
6. Top it with crushed almonds, some flaky sea salt and serve

Sauté Corn

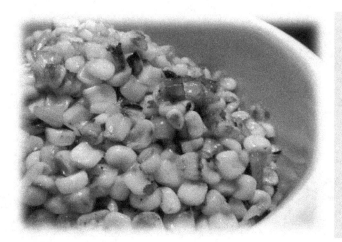

Time required:
25 minutes

Servings: 12

INGREDIENTS

10 eggs
1 cup cooked chicken, chopped
3 tbsp green onions, chopped
1/4 tsp garlic powder
Pepper Salt

STEPS FOR COOKING

1. Preheat the oven to 400 F.
2. Spray a muffin tray with cooking spray and set aside.
3. In a large bowl, whisk eggs with garlic powder, pepper, and salt.
4. Add remaining ingredients and stir well.
5. Pour egg mixture into the muffin tray and bake for 15 minutes.
6. Serve and enjoy.

Sweet Potatoes with Coconut

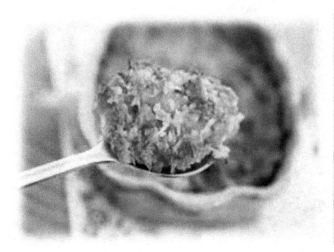

Time required:
60 minutes

Servings: 08

INGREDIENTS	STEPS FOR COOKING

4 nice, sliced potatoes

A sprinkling of olive oil

1 tiny community of thyme, chopped

1/3 cup of cream with coconut

1/2 parsley tsp., minced

1 tablespoon of Mustard Dijon

1/2 teaspoon of garlic

1. On a rimmed baking sheet, organize sweet potato slices, drizzle oil, spray thyme, season with a touch of salt and black pepper, mix properly, place at 400 degrees F in the oven, and bake for about 1 hour.

2. In the meantime, combine the coconut cream with the parsley, garlic, and mustard in a bowl and stir well together.

3. On trays, organize baked potatoes, sprinkle the mustard sauce all over, and serve as a side dish.

Chorizo and Egg Tortilla

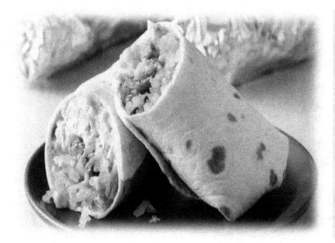

Time required:
25 minutes

___

Servings: 01

INGREDIENTS

1 flour tortilla, about 6-inches
1/3 cup chorizo meat, chopped 1 egg

STEPS FOR COOKING

1. Take a medium-sized skillet pan, place it over medium heat and when hot, add chorizo.

2. When the meat has cooked, drain the excess fat, whisk an egg, pour it into the pan, stir until combined, and cook for 3 minutes, or until eggs have cooked.

3. Spoon egg onto the tortilla and then serve.

Beer Pork Ribs

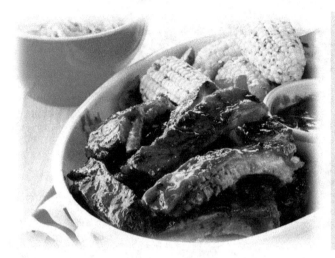

Time required:
8 hours

Servings: 01

INGREDIENTS

into two units/racks
18 oz. of root beer
2 cloves of garlic,
minced
2 tbsp. of onion
powder
2 tbsp. of vegetable
oil (optional)

STEPS FOR COOKING

1. Wrap the pork ribs with vegetable oil and place one unit on the bottom of your slow cooker with half of the minced garlic and the onion powder.

2. Place the other rack on top with the rest of the garlic and onion powder.

3. Pour over the root beer and cover the lid.

4. Let simmer for 8 hours on low heat.

5. Take off and finish optionally in a grilling pan for a nice sear.

Roasted Zucchini

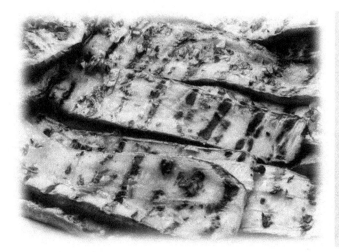

Time required:
35 minutes

Servings: 04

INGREDIENTS

1 lb. Zucchini, sliced
1 oz parmesan
cheese, grated
1 tsp dried mix herbs
1 garlic clove,
minced
2 tbsp olive oil

STEPS FOR COOKING

1. Preheat the oven to 450 f/ 232 c. Add all ingredients except parmesan cheese into the large bowl and toss well.

2. Transfer the zucchini mixture to the baking dish and cook in preheated oven for 10 minutes. Sprinkle parmesan cheese over zucchini.

3. Return to the oven and cook for 5 minutes more.

4. Serve and enjoy.

Tomato Mozzarella Salad

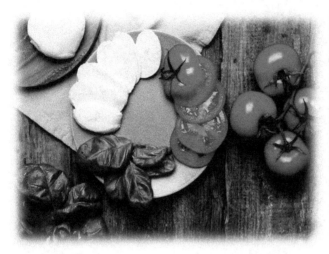

Time required:
15 minutes

Servings: 06

INGREDIENTS

5 medium tomatoes
1 bunch of fresh
basil leaves
½ teaspoon cracked
black pepper
2 cups apple cider
vinegar
¼ cup olive oil
32-ounce logs of
fresh mozzarella
cheese, full-fat

STEPS FOR COOKING

1. Cut tomato and cheese into ½-inch
   thick slices and then arrange these
   slices with basil in an alternating
   pattern in two rows in a small
   casserole dish.

2. Drizzle with oil and vinegar and
   season with salt and black pepper.

Garlic Soup

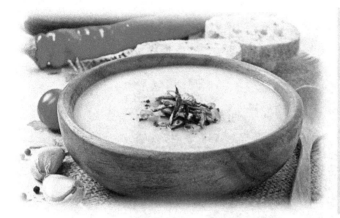

Time required:
15 minutes

___

Servings: 02

INGREDIENTS

5 cups water
Head garlic,
unpeeled Sprigs
fresh thyme
2 Tablespoons
further virgin olive
oil
Salt
Freshly ground black
pepper
2 egg yolks
Slices of bread,
gently toasted

STEPS FOR COOKING

1. Bring the water to boil with the garlic and thyme and simmer for twenty minutes.

2. Take away the garlic and peel. Place the flesh in an exceedingly bowl and mash with a fork.

3. Step by step add the vegetable oil and blend well. Return to the soup.

4. Take away the thyme and after that you should season it with salt & black pepper.

5. Beat the egg yolks in another bowl and step by step add a ladleful of the soup.

6. Combine well and stir into the soup. Simmer for some minutes, however don't let it boil or the soup can curdle.

7. Place the slices of toasts in individual bowls and pour over the soup. Serve at once.

Lemon Mousse

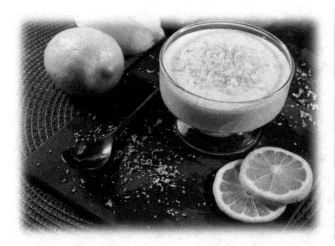

Time required:
25 minutes

Servings: 04

INGREDIENTS

1 cup coconut cream

8 Oz cream cheese, soft

¼ cup fresh lemon juice

3 pinches salt

1 tsp lemon liquid stevia

STEPS FOR COOKING

1. Preheat your oven to 350 °F.
2. Grease a ramekin with butter.
3. Beat cream, cream cheese, fresh lemon juice, salt and lemon liquid stevia in a mixer.
4. Pour batter into ramekin.
5. Bake for 10 minutes, then transfer the mousse to a serving glass.
6. Let it chill for 2 hours and serve. Enjoy!

Easy Fudge

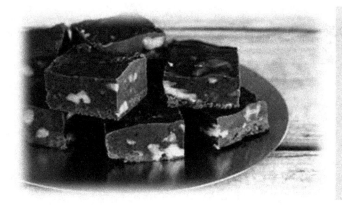

Time required:
45 minutes

Servings: 12

INGREDIENTS

1¾ cups of coconut
butter
1 cup pumpkin
puree
1 tsp ground
cinnamon
¼ tsp ground
nutmeg
1tbsp coconut oil

STEPS FOR COOKING

1. Take an 8x8 inch square baking pan and line it with aluminum foil.
2. Take a spoon and scoop out the coconut butter into a heated pan and allow the butter to melt.
3. Keep stirring well and remove from the heat once fully melted.
4. Add spices and pumpkin and keep straining until you have a grain-like texture.
5. Add coconut oil and keep stirring to incorporate everything distribute it. Scoop the mixture into your baking pan and evenly.
6. Place wax paper on top of the mixture and press gently tostraighten the top.
7. Remove the paper and discard.
8. Allow it to chill for 1-2 hours.
9. Once chilled, take it out and slice it up into pieces. Enjoy!

Homemade Granola

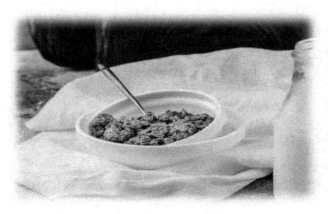

Time required:
55 minutes

Servings: 08

INGREDIENTS

*4 tablespoons of
vegetable oil or
sunflower oil
1 lemon juice table
spoon
2 tablespoons of
brown soft sugar
2 tablespoons clear
honey or golden
syrup Dried
cranberries
(optional)
300g (10½oz) rolled
oats*

STEPS FOR COOKING

1. Preheat the oven to 140 ° C (120 ° C
   Fan)/275 ° F / Gas 1.

2. The oil, syrup/honey, lemon juice and
   sugar are melted in a large saucepan
   over a low heat. The intention is not
   to allow the mixture to bubble, only to
   allow the ingredients to melt and
   blend together. Then add the oats and
   stir thoroughly.

3. Spread the mixture in an even layer
   on a baking tray (depending on their
   size, you will need two baking trays.
   Bake in the oven until crisp for around
   30-40 minutes. Check the granola
   every ten minutes and stir to ensure
   an even bake.

4. You can add a few handfuls of dried
   cranberries once cooked and cooled.
   The granola should be kept in an
   airtight container and utilized within
   one month.

Coffee Brownies

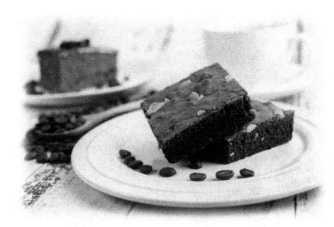

Time required:
45 minutes

Servings: 04

INGREDIENTS

3 eggs, beaten
2 tablespoons cocoa powder
2 teaspoons Erythritol
½ cup almond flour
½ cup organic almond milk

STEPS FOR COOKING

1. Place the eggs in the mixing bowl and combine them with Erythritol and almond milk.
2. With the help of the hand mixer, whisk the liquid until homogenous.
3. Then add almond flour and cocoa powder.
4. Whisk the mixture until smooth.
5. Take the non-sticky brownie mold and transfer the cocoa mass inside it.
6. Flatten it gently with the help of the spatula. The flattened mass should be thin.
7. Preheat the oven to 365 °F.
8. Transfer the brownie to the oven and bake it for 20 minutes.
9. Then chill the cooked brownies at least till room temperature and cut into serving bars.

Dessert Cocktail

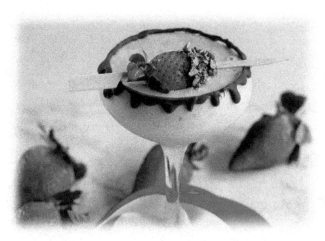

Time required:
5 minutes

Servings: 02

INGREDIENTS

1 cup of cranberry juice

1 cup of fresh ripe strawberries, washed and hull removed

2 tablespoon of lime juice

¼ cup of white sugar

8 ice cubes

STEPS FOR COOKING

1. Toss all ingredients in a blender until smooth and creamy.
2. Pour the liquid into chilled tall glasses and serve cold.

Apple Crunch Pie

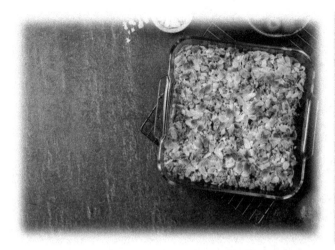

Time required:
45 minutes

Servings: 08

INGREDIENTS	STEPS FOR COOKING

4 large tart apples, peeled, seeded and sliced

½ cup of white all-purpose flour

1/3 cup margarine

1 cup of sugar

¾ cup of rolled oat flakes

½ teaspoon of ground nutmeg

1. Preheat the oven to 375F/180C.
2. Place the apples over a lightly greased square pan (around 7 inches).
3. Mix the rest of the ingredients in a medium bowl with and spread the batter over the apples.
4. Bake for about 30-35 minutes, until the top crust has gotten golden brown.
5. Serve hot.

Tart Apple Granita

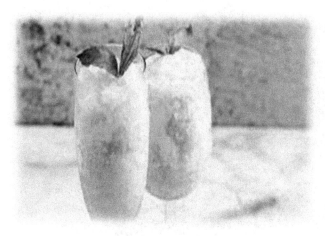

Time required:
15 minutes

Servings: 04

INGREDIENTS	STEPS FOR COOKING

INGREDIENTS

½ cup granulated sugar

½ cup water

2 cups unsweetened apple juice

¼ cup freshly squeezed lemon juice

STEPS FOR COOKING

1. Heat the sugar and water.
2. Bring to a boil and then lessen the heat to low and simmer for about 15 minutes or until the liquid has reduced by half.
3. Take away the pan from the heat and pour the liquid into a large shallow metal pan.
4. Let the liquid cool for about 40 minutes and then stir in the apple juice and lemon juice.
5. Place the pan in the freezer.
6. After 1 hour, run a fork through the liquid to break up any ice crystals formed. Scrape down the sides as well.
7. Place the pan back in the freezer and repeat the stirring and scraping every 20 minutes, creating slush.

INGREDIENTS	STEPS FOR COOKING
	8. Serve when the mixture is completely frozen and looks like crushed ice, after about 3 hours.

CPSIA information can be obtained
at www.ICGtesting.com
Printed in the USA
BVHW090534220621
610124BV00011B/2608

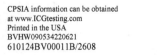

9 781802 611281